I0410493

And Then There Were Six
A Mother's Diary

By

Teri Hirsch

© 2003 by Teri Hirsch. All rights reserved.

No part of this book may be reproduced, stored in a
retrieval system, or transmitted by any means, electronic,
mechanical, photocopying, recording, or otherwise, without
written permission from the author.

ISBN: 1-4033-9452-0 (e-book)
ISBN: 1-4033-9453-9 (Paperback)

This book is printed on acid free paper.

1stBooks – rev. 12/18/02

Prelude

When we are young we are all so sure of what we want in life, that many of us are truly confident that we will get it by sheer will. Many even have ideas of who the perfect person is that we will marry, how old we will be (or at least want to be) when certain events happen in our lives, where we will live and what we will be doing for a living. You may gain some control over these things but when you sit down to think about it, no one really knows ahead of time what life will bring them. So much of life involves your current surroundings, your present financial situation, your location, your community, the people in our life and most of all, that very special *someone else.* Today's wants and needs may change with tomorrow's decisions. Unfortunately, it is hard to find out that there are no givens in life. Yet, that is what makes life interesting.

Take, for instance, the ability to conceive children. The majority of people, even today, still take for granted their ability to have children. Reality, however, is that for far more people than you may think, having children is not a given. Sometimes people have to try to come to terms with what God has dealt them. Thankfully, modern medical research has been able to find numerous ways to help people out who might not otherwise have had the opportunity to bear children. It is these parents who have worked so hard that truly appreciate the gift that has been given them. May we all have the honor of being able to feel such gratitude in our lives.

After discovering that there were some couples we knew personally that were in such a predicament, my husband's and my understanding of the value of children in our lives became very apparent. At this time we were making a decision of our own on the subject of children, our decision was to try for a large family, even with such preliminary thoughts, we still did not know whether or not it was going to be easy or hard. We, like millions of others, put the negative possibilities in the far reaches of our minds. Again, like so many, we said to ourselves that those things happen to "them" not us. Only difference this time was that we knew the "them".

We did make one other decision, that after we had exhausted all options (if we had to) we would consider adoption. There was something about a large family that appealed to both of us. So on we went to try.

Fortunately for us our fears were never met, we were blessed with the ability to have more fun than trouble in conceiving our children. The following stories will hopefully give you some insights to some real pregnancies and the things that can happen, not necessarily the things you read about in cold textbooks.

There is a multitude of changes going on in your body during pregnancy that are out of your control and yet are perfectly normal. Anything from your physical appearance to your mental health can change in the blink of an eye, or so it feels. These are not necessarily the things your doctor tells you about until you ask. One very good reason for that is that there are *so many* variations of each of these changes that it would take a doctor more time to tell you about them than it would for you to have the baby. Your doctor will wait for your questions as the need arises, he/she may even ask you if you have questions or concerns during each visit. *So don't be afraid to ask.* The information and stories you have heard from your friends or mothers regarding their pregnancy doesn't mean you will nor does it mean the same event will affect you the same way either. It is possible to experience totally new things with each subsequent child. Each child is someone completely different and therefore, it stands to reason that each pregnancy could potentially affect you in completely different ways. This is something I found out the hard way.

One item that I can not stress enough is that it is very important to *know your own body* ahead of time. This way if something feels amiss, you'll know right away. Check it out, it's only a phone call, the doctors are expecting to hear from you.

Often times you will find an obstetricians' office has nurse practitioners working there as well, they are there to help you, they are qualified in answering most of your questions and if they can't they will get back to you with what the doctor wants you to do. Having open communication between you and your doctor during this time is <u>very crucial, he/she can't read your mind</u>. There is equal if not more value in discussing your mental or physical concerns with your husband/partner as well. Don't leave him out, he too can be a source of continuous support if you let him.

From one child to the next, I still had questions to ask. Certain things stayed the same, while still other issues came up I never experienced before. I am hoping that the following stories will help you see just how different one person's pregnancies can be. I went through each one, each with their own set of ups and downs, and most importantly, each with the help of a great doctor's practice and a loving, supportive husband.

For many, reading about what can possibly happen is very calming, it helps them to understand that what is going on with them, is not unique and that they are not alone. For others it makes them worry. Don't worry, your doctors and nurses are there to help you through it all. It is my hope for you that you also have a great support group, be it family or friends. Again I can't emphasize enough that you should know your own body. Know where you are starting from so that you know when there are changes and if they are extreme or not. Know if you have weaknesses in certain places – ask your doctor if pregnancy will affect them. I did, I have rheumatoid arthritis, not a debilitating disease but a chronic one nonetheless. As it turned out, the doctor said that many times during pregnancy the type of arthritis that I have can be kicked into a kind of remission. I was relieved to hear that it won't affect the baby in any way. All I had to do was to stop my medication.

Other medical conditions; such as diabetes, hypothyroid, kidney disease, liver disease, high blood pressure or any other such conditions should be discussed before even becoming pregnant. For people with any of these conditions or any other chronic illnesses, specialists may need to be involved before, during, and after the pregnancy as well. Take care of yourself the right way, you want this baby to have a mother who is healthy enough to keep up with them not one who needs as much care as the infant does. Be smart, check out everything. It would be a good suggestion, that if you have never been to a OBGYN before that you may want to do so even before you get pregnant so that he/she can see where you are starting from, your blood pressure, your iron count, etc... These are all important factors in being pregnant.

Sorry I digress. Yes, we have been blessed with the ability to have children. We did not get this far without some turbulence. Truth is, I am sure there are many people out there who would say my version of turbulence is nothing compared to what they had. I am not denying that it could have been worse, I'm just telling you what happened to me. My pregnancies were each as different as the personalities of the children they involved, and so were the deliveries.

Do not let what you are about to read scare you, just think of it as food for thought. I am not writing this so that you can get all the answers either, that's for your doctor to answer, I just would like to let you know that there is someone out there that understands what you are about to go through or already went through and that there is someone out there that cares enough to tell you—you can do this, you have the power within you to withstand anything pregnancy will give you. Please also remember that there is icing on this cake and it is one of natures finest.

Chapter 1

Our first child was on the way. As with many first time moms, it seemed to me that this whole pregnancy thing was going to be no big deal. Everyone kept referring to the phrase of how a pregnant woman has a glow about her. That it brings joy to everyone around. Everything I kept hearing portrayed only the positives images of what people remember about pregnancy, or what "they have always heard", not necessarily the realities.

I had a good job, a loving and supportive husband, wonderful family all around, I was expecting our first child, life was good, what could be so bad about this? I was about to find out.

So far everything was fine, I didn't have to deal with any cramps that month, I didn't have to carry anything extra with me at all times. I wasn't sure just what was so tough about this whole thing. So, I was going to gain some weight and possibly some more hormonal attitude. Then it hit me, *the nausea*. Every night, at least three times a night, I was jolted awake with an astounding wave of nausea that told me I had to do something NOW! It would come upon me in my sleep, being a light sleeper didn't' help at all. I wonder, thinking back, that if I was a heavier sleeper maybe it wouldn't have awoken me, or maybe it would have awoken me too late. I guess we'll never know.

It was beginning to feel that my body was connected to the lunar clock and the nausea would just show up as the sun went down. To be perfectly fine one minute and the next have the overwhelming feeling that you needed to throw up, was quite frustrating. Oh, maybe I should mention that the thing I have always hate most about being sick is being nauseated. So I'm sure you can't even imagine my comfort level during these episodes mainly because I don't think there are even words for it.

There were no warning signs at all, not even a progression of activity just an instantaneous nausea. My biggest frustration became trying to figure out when it was coming and how long was it going to last. Many nights I was even afraid to eat dinner, I had to force myself because otherwise I would then feel guilty that I was not feeding the child. What a horrible feeling – like your not a good mother when the baby wasn't even close to being born.

Needless to say, the first 3 months or so I went to sleep with a full package of salty crackers and some kind of white soda next to my bed, only to finally wake in the morning to see it all gone. Salty things are the one thing that I have found to be consistently helpful in soothing my nausea. I didn't always remember getting up during the night, but obviously I did.

After the first 6 weeks or so my nightly visits became more frequent. Friends, family, the books and the doctor all mentioned something called "morning sickness" but no one warned me how often "morning" came. Nothing I remember reading talked about "morning" being at 7 am 10 am, 2pm, 5pm, 9pm etc... you get the picture. The waves of nausea were still coming without warning, unfortunately for me the only thing that would calm down my stomach and head was when I would eat. (A salt and water diet? Gee, you think I was retaining water?) I guess eating every time was better than throwing up each time, I had been told that that could have happened as well. As a matter of fact, I have friends that actually lost weight during the first couple of months because of the amount of times they actually threw up. Maybe if I threw up it would have been better than being in a, what seemed to be, permanent state of nausea.

No it's not a pretty picture, but this is the single most common "ailment" of pregnancy, I am told. It has to do with the tremendous hormone changes your body is going through. It sounds like a simple thing that can easily be taken care of, people on television shows make fun of it all the time. Yet, for some people, it's not so simple, and surely not so funny.

Some people say it has to do with how much the baby is like the mother. The more things different the more the body will react. I don't know if there is really any scientific proof behind this though. As with anything that involves your body, this too can become a serious thing, this is one of those things that if it gets to an extreme amount, if you find yourself getting weak because of it or lightheaded – *call the doctor*. An adult can dehydrate a lot quicker than you might think, especially if you are vomiting too much.

If you are the type of person that vomits, please talk it over with your doctor as to what he/she recommends you do if it gets too severe. Ask how you are to tell if it is getting worse. There are some things that he/she can suggest you do. Don't get paranoid into thinking that if you throw up more than once a week you will dehydrate, use your head and decide for yourself at what point you would like to call, or ask ahead of time how much is too much and what should you do. Asking a question is not being a nuisance, however, not asking can lead to trouble.

Remember when you were back in school and the teacher said, "the only dumb question is the one you don't ask". I can't express enough how important it is to be open and honest with your doctor. Sure they have heard these question before, but not from you, and the only way they can truly be helpful during this pregnancy is if you let them know what is going on.

But I digress, again. After those first three months things seemed to calm down in the nausea department. Then came the curse, at least according to my grandmother it was anyway. For any of you who can do math, try this one on for *size,* I started out the pregnancy wearing a DD cup bra, by the time I was nursing the baby I was three number sizes bigger plus an F cup. This was *not* something I bargained for. Sure I heard that your chest will grow somewhat during pregnancy and again when you had the baby if you plan on nursing, but 6 full sizes different was another story!! Being only 5'1" you can imagine how hard it was to carry this around. It felt that every other month if not sooner I had to go into a new lingerie place to get the next size up.

To add insult to injury, my stomach was growing at an alarming rate (in my view). There was only an inch or two between the bottom of my bra and the top of my skirts.

When I looked in the mirror I felt like the little girl in the Willie Wonka and the Chocolate Factory movie, you know the one, the one who ate the gum and blew up like a giant blueberry and had to be rolled out of the room. No one warned me that ones self image could be crushed.

Why did I have to keep finding new places? First off, I felt a little embarrassed. Second though was a little harder to take, with each new place I would receive the same response, "Oh honey, you can't need that big – you're so short" then when I would put one on, the size I told them in the first place, the response would always be, "wow, I wouldn't believe it if I didn't see it for myself". As if trying on a new sized bra in front of a perfect stranger wasn't hard enough, the comments I could have done without. These women were supposedly "professional". One time in particular I remember that when I walked out of the store I looked over my shoulder and saw the sales clerk pointing me out and talking to someone else. Once or twice I saw it happening while I was still in the store, I felt like a freak, when all I was, was a pregnant person with overactive mammary glands. They sold the sizes, surely they had to have sold them to someone before. Don't you think?

As round as I felt my stomach was getting, my chest was having a contest to see who could reach the next room first. I realized even then that this was no health hazard and doing no harm to the baby. Sure I understood that one's bust size would increase, but the self-conscious part wasn't in the books, they only talked about this supposed wonderful "glow" of an expectant mother. I was not glowing, only growing. This obviously doesn't happen to every person who starts off with a large chest, but I'm positive that I'm not the only one either. Unfortunately, for the person going through it, it's hard to feel you have any company at all.

There was some humor used to defuse the depression part of it. We were once at my in-laws and everyone around the table was asking me if I was planning on nursing the baby or not. My husband insisted that we were having twins, just on my sheer size, it's not like he had any backing from the doctors. Just to egg my husband on more someone asked me how I would nurse twins. Without hesitation, and from only listening from the other room, my husband yells out, "Don't worry, *my* wife can." Maybe it was at that point that I was actually glowing, only it was out of embarrassment not pregnancy.

Then something wonderful started to happen. The baby started moving enough so that we could feel it. There are no words to describe how one feels the first time you feel the life you have created. Every negative feeling you may have had up until now has all been pushed by the way side only to be replaced with sheer exhilaration and anticipation of feeling the movement again.

Toward the end of the fifth month and on there was one thing I truly looked forward to every night. That was my baby's nightly dancing. Actually, it was more rolling than anything else. This baby would start on one side and push out, then in a slow gradual movement as if it was turning over, you would see that bump go from the left side of my belly to the center and back down on the right side and sometimes back again.

On one occasion I remember my husband said, he didn't believe it, he thought I was forcing this to happen. Until the time when I held my hands up and he put his hands on top of this rolling ball. I can only tell you that when you first begin to feel the child move inside of you everything else in the world becomes irrelevant, at least for that moment. It is with this that you remember why you started this to begin with. Often times it is the mobility of the baby that begins to make the pregnancy a joint venture. Frequently husbands/partners like to massage the belly to stimulate the baby so they can share in the experience, as for the mother, well, who wouldn't want a massage? This event makes the pregnancy real for your "other half".

Round and round we grew where she'll stop nobody knows. The baby was getting busier and busier. Sometimes I would purposely put something on my stomach, like the remote control to see how long it would take for it to be rolled off. The best was when the baby would get hic-cups and whatever you put there would have this steady hop to it.

Nobody I know personally gets through a pregnancy without a couple of pitfalls, in the scheme of things, this first pregnancy went well. Towards the end, we wanted to be prepared for the inevitable birth. So we took Lamaze classes. Our instructor was of the opinion that you reduce fears through the education of what will be happening in your body and what each stage means. I highly recommend these types of classes to any first -time parents. Refresher courses aren't bad either if there has been a long time between children.

Memorial Day, Monday 6:30 am, I felt something pop inside me and made a dart towards the bathroom. Whew! I made it - my water had broken. The flush of water that comes out is incredible, for some reason I wasn't expecting so much. Then again, being the first I wasn't sure what to expect. All excited, I came out with only enough time to tell my husband the baby was coming. Then there was more water. We talked to the doctor, he said congratulations, and I will see you later. We now had to wait until the contractions would get closer and/or until I was at the point that I could not talk through one.

Only a half an hour later and the contractions started. Although the classes as well as the doctor told us that they would start far apart and get closer, my child decided to do things differently. From 7 am until I went to the hospital at 4:30 pm my contractions came every 5-7 minutes. By the time we arrived at the hospital I was in such intense pain that I did not know what was going on inside me. I had to try really hard to refocus. In some strange way, just being there and assuming that things were near an end I was able to calm down.

Unfortunately for me the doctor didn't come until 7 pm (twelve hours after the labor pains had started). The interns at the hospital had reported to the doctor that I wasn't having very hard contractions. Maybe not to them, they weren't feeling a thing.

Anyway, when he did finally come, he did what's called an internal exam to see just how far dilated I was. Dilation is determined in centimeters and is the measurement of the hole in which your cervix has opened to in order for the birthing process to take place. Full dilation is at 10 centimeters.

After all this time I was not very far along, only 4 centimeters it was decided that my contractions were going to have to be much stronger in order to move the baby down, yet it had also already been 12 hours. This doctor helped us to make the decision to go ahead with the drug called an epidural. It is administered in the women's spine to alleviate pain and pressure felt in the back and in the pelvis area. It was only after it had been administered that we realized all this time I had been experiencing what is known as back labor. The first contraction after that, I remember as not being so bad and understood why the doctor said they would have to be stronger.

Along with this, the baby was not dropping into the position it needed to be in order to move down through what is called the birthing canal, so the doctor gave me another intravenous drug called potosin to help move things along. It also makes your contractions stronger.

I remember watching the monitors and seeing that the nurse and/or the doctor kept increasing the potosin because the baby was still way too high. They were also concerned about the fact that the water broke so many hours prior to this. Things moved along, just not very fast, I was not up to pushing the baby out until 10:30 pm, 16 hours after my contraction started.

When I was pushing, I made the mistake of using my facial muscles too much and not enough of my abdominal muscles. Of course, at the time I didn't realize this, it was only afterwards when you saw how my face looked from the broken blood vessels (very freckled) that you knew. By 11:07 pm the baby was born.

The baby's cord was cut and then it was swooped away from us, before we knew it there was a team of doctors and nurses using all kinds of things to attend to the baby with, we didn't even know what sex the baby was yet. The doctor told us that a tremendous flush of meconium (baby's first stool) went over her face and they needed to make sure the baby did not inhale any of this. After they determined that things were stable and the baby was out of danger, we found out – It's a girl! 8 lb 1 oz.

What about the weight you ask? Those 40 some odd pounds I gained? Well all I can say is only 3 weeks later, 25 were lost already. I told you there was a lot of water. This was really comforting to me. Never having been overweight by more than 10 pounds, pregnancy can really do a number on your ego. Sure you know why you're gaining, still the numbers can bother you.

How long would it take for my body to get back on track was my next concern. Oddly though, it only took about 2 ½ months after she was born for my period to come back. I was so surprised, I thought the post pardum bleeding was starting all over again, or maybe I was hemorrhaging, but when I called the doctor, he said, "It's just your period, carry on as usual." So much for the old wives tale that you can't get pregnant while nursing. I guess that only applies for the women who don't get their period during nursing. In some way, however, it was quite comforting to know that my body was "back to normal".

My pediatrician of that time gave me a "formula" in which to use to help determine how much the baby should eat on each side, how long etc... The advice changed with each baby, so the best advice I can give you is to talk to your pediatrician and ask him/her what they think. Or ask a lactation specialist. Many hospitals provide them, ask for one while you are still in the hospital. They will give you all the information you need to make your nursing experience a good one.

I could go on for a year about how cute she was but that is not why we are here is it?

Chapter 2

When the baby was only 4 months old we figured out that the only advantage to getting back your period early is that you know when you miss one. Not being a hundred percent sure why my period was late, I called the doctor. To be safe he wanted me to come in for some blood work. When I went in the doctor said that famous phrase, "I have good news and bad news."

The good news? I was pregnant. So what could he possibly say is the bad news?? That I had to give up nursing the baby. Why you ask? Quite simply it was when he showed me a menu of what I would have to eat in order to supply enough nutrients to the nursing baby, the growing baby and myself, I almost threw up. The lesser of the two evils was to stop nursing. I left the office with very mixed feelings. I didn't want to deny my baby of mother's milk and yet I didn't want to deprive the new one of anything either. However, I didn't think it was possible for me to eat as much as was necessary.

My first big problem was thinking I knew what to do. It never even crossed my mind to ask the doctor how to stop nursing. Needless to say, being naive and stupid (emphasis on the stupid) I stopped nursing cold turkey. The baby was already getting some bottles anyway, she wouldn't mind. Taking a bottle was easier than nursing for the baby because it was less work for her. This was not a child that particularly loved nursing or cuddling. It seemed that the only person who did mind going cold turkey was me. Whoa!!!! No one told me your breasts would become so engorged that they would be hard as rocks until your body finally figured out you were no longer nursing and it had to stop producing milk. OOOOOOOOWWWWWWWW!!! Ok, so I learned that lesson real quick – always wean off.

Certain old fashion ideas really work. Of course, afterwards I was told how it all works. One of the many miracles of having children is that your body also learns how much milk to produce for the baby based on how much he/she eats. It will continue to produce this much until you wean the baby off to the point that you are no longer nursing. Only after this does your body "know" when to stop its milk production. Ok, so the body is smarter than the mind. Gee, I wonder how that works?

What I did was plain dumb. My body was still producing at full speed ahead only I put a cork on the bottle, the pressure really built up. Numerous hot showers and heating pads later I was finally able to hug the baby and not be in pain. In truth it only took about 3-4 days of being totally uncomfortable, then things started to get back to normal. The good news is that my size was shrinking, even being pregnant with the next one. It was as if my body wanted to start from the beginning again.

The children were going to be 13 months apart. One of my biggest concerns was that I would be carrying around two babies at the same time – all the time. Thankfully my "miss independent" decided to learn how to walk on her own by 10 months. Which means there would be 3 full months before the baby was born, plenty of time for her to master walking.

With this baby I had to change my doctor in the middle, we had moved and I had to find someone right away being already 4½ months pregnant. One of the first things this new doctor talked to me about was that I had already passed the time of when they do a routine ultrasound. He offered to do it anyway if I wanted it. I decided that it wasn't necessary since I had done fine without it the first time. I did mention that I was not objecting to it however, if he ever felt that I needed it I would have been happy to do it.

My first doctor did not use an ultrasound regularly. He felt that it should only be used when medically necessary and not just to check to see if the baby was there.

Here is another example why talking to friends and relatives can give you conflicting information. They all could have gone to a different doctor, therefore, they were instructed to do things in slightly different ways. None of which were wrong, only different.

If you have the time before you get pregnant, interview some doctors to find out if they offer the options that you would want either during your pregnancy or during the birthing process. If you disagree with a doctor's philosophy on what you consider to be major issues, don't use them, find someone who you trust more, it's your body and your baby and you have the right to pick a doctor who will help and guide you through a pregnancy and birth the way you feel the most comfortable.

There I go again, sorry. This time I wanted to beat the nausea train, so I had my saltines and soda prepared every night, and yet the train never came to my station. Believe me when I say, I didn't miss having it. My other fear was halted when my chest stopped growing by the sixth month and it wasn't nearly as large. As it turned out I was gaining only a fraction of the weight that I did previously. By the end of the 2nd trimester last pregnancy I was already past the 30 pound mark, now I was only around 20 pounds. This makes a big difference, especially when you have someone else to run after.

One of the most notable differences between the two pregnancies was the way they moved. As I said in the beginning of the book, my pregnancies were as different as the children themselves. This one, for instance, kicked and punched, no smooth rolls to be found. All day and especially at night I could feel the punches and jabs from this one. Sometimes this baby would kick and leave its foot pressed up on my stomach in a stretch and hold that we could have sworn we saw the shape of a foot.

For the child already here, however, every time she wanted to hold mommy, she received a punch or kick too. For awhile she would kick me back not understanding what was going on. We did tell her there was a baby inside reaching out to her to meet her, but she was still a baby herself and the concept was just too much for her. She would still express how upset she was with me whenever it happened.

When my daughter would fall asleep on me, she was certain to be jarred awake by a nudge or a bump. I am sure you can just imagine how well this was received.

To take the edge off of being kicked in the face we taught her the game of putting things on top of mommy's belly to watch the baby kick it off. This would keep her entertained for quit a long time. The down side to this was that I had to have the time to sit and do it. Mommy's patience usually wore out before her desire to quit the game was there. One time when I had to stand up and answer the phone, she said to me, "baby not done mommy". I had to gently tell her that may be true but mommy was.

When the time came, it was once again, early morning. Approximately 5:30 am to be more precise. My husband was in the shower he came out to see me rubbing my back. My children just love that spot in my back and feel this incredible need to snuggle up against it during labor.

After the first hour or so we realized this time that it was back labor,.... Again. We called the doctor immediately to say that we would like to get to the hospital sooner than later. I didn't want to go through another 12, hours like last time, of back pain. The next phone call was to my in-laws to come and watch my daughter because we had to leave. They came with smiles on, my daughter had gotten up just in time to see them come in. It phased her not that we were leaving, the grandparents were here, and she could have them all day we told her.

Everything seemed to be on super speed mode. When we first arrived in the hospital, I was expecting my water to break any second and it did not. In fact, the doctor found, through the internal exam, that I was already 7 centimeters (out of 10) dilated. In other words, the baby was coming fast. After spending an entire day in labor last time, I wasn't ready for this, mentally anyway.

So close and so little time had passed, it was only around 10 am, only about 5 hours had passed. Yes, I am not ashamed to say that I needed to take the epidural again anyway. However, they only gave me enough to take the edge off my back. They wanted to insure that I was able to feel the contractions so that I could tell when it was time to push the baby out. It's very important to have some feeling, they told me.

Using the epidural is not a cop-out nor should it be thought of as such, especially for someone like me who seemed to be having large children who loved to push on your back. Also, not knowing how long this one was going to take, I had to get some relief on my back. If you have never know the pain of back labor the only way I can describe it to you is to compare it to a kidney stone (which I have also had). If you haven't had either one - good for you. The force of a baby's head, muscle contractions and the speed that this one was moving made for an intensity on my back that is immeasurable. It was as if each contraction also squeezed out my tears, they just kept coming.

At this point the doctor had to break the water for me because it didn't want to go on its own. How does it feel to sit in a bed and have a balloon full of warm water popped under you? Yech! It's warm, its gooey and it's now all over you. My first thought was, when do I get to shower? It actually relieves some of the pressure and yet it also increases the amount you feel the baby move, and this baby was ready to move. Each contraction after this was a lot more intense because there was no water to cushion the pressure. Besides my little baby kick and punch was as active as ever, kicking or banging into anything in its path.

Time passed quickly enough that we hardly had time to notice the clock, before we knew it this baby was ready to come out, it was time to push, still after only a few pushes I found myself to be at a point of sheer exhaustion and couldn't push anymore. I was drained of energy, I couldn't figure out why I was so tired when it wasn't as long as the last one. But my body really wanted to rest. My head was pounding, my arms hurt from being tense and I felt as if I was fading in and out. Truthfully with all this going on I just wanted to give into the exhaustion and sleep. This one was a lot more work to push out.

The doctor said that I was only able to stop because of the medicine, otherwise I should have already pushed the baby out, they could see it already. The tone of his voice was that of a person who was impatient and needed to be somewhere else. This made me feel really guilty, like a quitter – I really was tired, my whole body was working so hard to get this baby out and here was a person telling me I was being lazy. There was no excuse for his tone of voice. I don't think I'll ever forget that. I felt awfully small at that moment.

It took only a couple more pushes and here came the monster that had been beating me up inside for so long. This one too had some meconium that came out but because it wasn't as large of a flush as was seen the last time, this doctor did not feel the need to have a whole team come to check out the baby.

The announcement finally came – a 9lb boy! And he wonders why I had trouble pushing it out? We were so overjoyed with emotion that we both had tears in our eyes. After working so hard the first time, I was too tired to be excited, and this time I was able somehow, to muster the strength.

As I had suspected, the doctor left as soon as I was stable. With all my excitement, this left a very bad taste in my mouth. Before he left he had only one comment to make, "The first was 8 this one is 9, I wonder what the next will be?" It was more sarcasm than humor. I was not amused.

My husband had left for the night to be with our daughter, and we had not seen the baby except for those first few minutes. The nurse came in to say the baby was still under the warmer because he was breathing too fast. She was very reassuring that this was normal in large babies. I took the opportunity to sleep a little, only to be interrupted by the pediatrician coming in to tell me that they needed to do a spinal tap on the baby.

Talk about a rude awakening. I practically fell over. The doctor explained that apparently the baby did inhale some of the miconium and they needed to check out his lungs for pneumonia, and any other complication that may have occurred due to this inhalation.

Around 1 am I had mustered up the strength to finally go see my baby in the intensive care unit. I have to admit, I was somewhat scared to go, I wasn't sure what to expect. There he was, so big that he practically filled one of those little bassinets with wires and things all over him, plus an oxygen bubble over his head. Next to him was a premature baby only about 3 ½ pounds, here he was the physical stature of a healthy baby and he looked just as pitiful as this little one next to him with the same tubes and monitors. It was quite disheartening. They let me touch him but everywhere you touched you felt wires not fresh soft skin.

I was unable to get hold of my husband that night, but when I finally spoke to him, he fell silent on the phone. He was expecting to hear how well the two of us were getting along, and instead I had other news to tell. He came right over to the hospital to see for himself what had transpired in his absence.

With all the possibilities of things that could go wrong, what happened to our son is actually considered rather mild. He was born on Friday so when Sunday came the hospital had to discharge me — he had to stay. I remember so distinctly being a real witch to everyone I saw that morning. My mother-in-law came with my daughter and I all but bit her head off. Of course, I apologized right away but with my emotions and hormones running amuck it was hard to control what came out of my mouth. My whole family, to this day, say they don't remember me being so bad, but I know exactly what I said that day. I also know exactly how I felt that day.

Leaving without the baby was like having your heart ripped out. I couldn't sleep, I called the nurse's station first thing in the morning. I have to admit though that they were quite understanding, and that they said I could come by any time I wanted to. Especially if I wanted to leave them some mother's milk for the baby. I went everyday, sometimes more than once. Using an electrical pump that the hospital provided was not something I was totally comfortable with either, but it was necessary. Imagine putting a plastic mask on your breast and watching yourself being "sucked" while the milk goes into a bottle. Yes, it is as weird as it sounds, and yes it looks as weird as it sounds. Essentially, I was being milked

With my permission and the permission of the other parents in the special care unit. My milk was used for anyone who needed it. It was not a problem for me to produce enough for the whole fraternity. At least that is what the nurses dubbed the nursery at the time, it was all boys.

My son came home a week later. Not a very long time in comparison to those we left behind, yet the emotional strain was still felt. And for the first month afterwards, I was still stopping by to check on my new friends. A couple of us stayed in touch for a few months. We all just needed an ear, this was before the internet was around. As far as I am aware all those boys went home healthy. This is where we can again say, thank God for modern medicine.

Chapter 3

We just can't get enough of their love. As I told you before, we were planning on a large family. We did wait a little longer on this one, these two were going to be 26 months apart. In fact by the time this one would be born, my first one would be starting nursery school.

This child was also the start of a new doctor. After experiencing the attitude of the last one, I was in no hurry to go back. Upon the recommendation of a close friend, I chose a new practice. What a difference a smile makes. In this new office, I was never greeted with less than a smile and a hello.

As I stated before, having a good, close relationship with your obstetrician is very important. It is much easier to establish a relationship when the people around you are all interested in your well being. This was such a place. The doctors, nurses and office staff all loved their jobs. The office, was decorated in light, friendly colors, flowers and plants throughout. Plus, plenty of women's health material written for the laymen to read and not a doctor's journal. Many of the magazines were helpful, they even had books for older soon-to-be siblings could read.

This office took the time to find out what we had been through before, they wanted to know everything so that he could asses any potential risks for future pregnancies. The nurse practitioner was also quite versed in my chart. I felt that as a team, I was in very good hands. Here was a group of people who loved what they do, how often can you say that?

My other children loved to go with me to the doctor's office. They found it fascinating to hear the baby's heartbeat. Standing on the scale was sometimes difficult though because they wanted to stand on it with me. The nurses there didn't mind when my kids came with me. They used to love to see how well the two of them got along. Truth is their giggles were contagious. Like most offices, within each patient's room there was a little "closet" with a curtain on it for you to change clothes in. The kids thought this was their own private secret cave.

During my first pregnancy our Lamaze instructor told us about the potential craving dangers you may experience during pregnancy. We couldn't imagine what she was talking about. The doctor had already given us a list of the most wild things that women have ingested because the craving was so strong.

Some of these things you wouldn't normally even equate with eating. Like laundry detergent because of the lemony smell. The "dangers" as they were referred to in class were classified as such because during your 7th month the vital organs are being formed and all the more so you should be careful not to give into an irrational craving.

Not having had any real cravings before that I couldn't ward off I never understood what the talk was all about. Then, here I was in the midst of my third pregnancy and her words came back to haunt me.

As a teenager I had smoked, but it had been over 10 years since then. Yet, the biggest craving I had was for nicotine. I caught myself walking closer to people who were smoking just to smell it. I saw myself go out of my way in the mall just to pass the store that sold the cigars and pipe tobacco.

My brother-in-law smoked and every time we were all together I used to go outside to talk to him while he smoked, and it wasn't for the company.

Then it hit me as to what I was doing. This is what she was talking about so many years ago. Nicotine is truly a "dangerous craving". It took a lot of strength and conscious behavior to overcome this craving. It wasn't easy sometimes, other times you realized the power of the craving would overtake the rational mind. I had to mention this to a couple of friends so that they would help me watch out for my own good. Thankfully, this lasted only about 6 weeks of off an on cravings. Who knew that something like that could come back to my life in such a strange form. I was relieved when this stage of my pregnancy was over.

With each pregnancy I sent a picture of myself, both front and side view, to my grandmother. She mulled over my shape, size, angle of belly – you name it and then she would decide whether I was going to have a girl or a boy. Problem was, she was wrong the first two times. It made her feel better knowing that I still valued her opinion though. I never reminded her what she had said either. She was pleased as punch that the fist two came out healthy. Boy or girl never really mattered to her. She was always more concerned about my health and the baby's well being. Oh, and that I would have enough milk to feed it. Amazing how long a little guilt will last in a person's heart.

As the summer went on carrying this extra weight wasn't making me too comfortable. For the last two my last trimester was in the spring, it wasn't too hot yet. This one was due in August and in my mind it was the hottest summer in New Jersey's history. Of course, if we would check the history books I'm sure I was wrong, but that's not how I felt. Humid, and sticky is not a good way to be pregnant. My natural body temperature had become increasingly intolerant to these weather conditions. I would walk around all day with a water bottle, some of it went into my mouth the rest on my head. The kids thought it was great fun, splashing mommy from the water in their little plastic pool. Warm pool water even felt good. But hey, things could have been worse.

I found myself showering sometimes twice a day. Thirst was another problem, I was never seen without a glass of water in my hand 24 hours a day 7 days a week. You can only imagine what drinking so much does for a pregnant women's bladder, and her weight.

Imagine my excitement though when I received an invitation to a friends wedding, then imagine how I felt when the date was within a week of my due date. Needless to say we responded that we would only be attending the ceremony. No need to pay for a meal for people who may have to leave early or not be there at all.

Our family likes to do things together. You see, at this time both of my sisters-in-law were pregnant as well. One was due three weeks after me and another four months later. We had a good time comparing our bellies. It was fun for the whole family.

Thankfully, there is not much to say about this pregnancy, pretty much everything went "by the book". The only exception was that this little one never stopped moving. When you go in for your check ups with the obstetrician, the doctor likes to hear the heartbeat of the baby. This time, it wasn't so easy. Only because this one felt an incredible need to move every time they would find it. Instead of the usual one or two minutes, it consistently took four or five minutes to get a good sound.

At this practice they routinely take an ultrasound early on to determine correct age of your baby. Considering that up until now I have not had one, I opted to forgo the ultrasound. The doctor was not thrilled but he understood why. He asked if it was a preference or an aversion. I explained that it was not an aversion but because I already went through pregnacies without it, I really didn't feel any great need to start something new.

Remember I told you about my friends wedding? Well, it was a good thing we responded we weren't going to be there. The day of my friend's wedding was a Sunday. A perfect day and a great time of day makes for a wonderful visit with the grandparents. They would baby-sit while we went to the ceremony. The hall was about a five minutes from their house. At least that was our original plan. The kids were all excited to spend the afternoon there, then we would come back and bring them home just in time to go to sleep.

The best laid plans aren't necessarily the ones that work the smoothest. Shortly before we were about to leave our house the contractions started. At first I was not too worried because I was having so many mild contractions for the past month, I didn't give these much of a thought. By the time we arrived at my in-laws house, only a half of an hour later. The story was different. I realized that this time it was not a false labor.

I'll never forget the look on my father-in-law's face. I was sitting on the couch, my husband on an easy chair, the kids were playing with toys, when they walked in. "Why aren't you guys getting dressed?" he asked "My wife is in labor." My husband said. "Why are you on my couch?!" my father-in-law asked. If only I had a camera at that moment. It was a cross between fear, anxiety and excitement – what a look! The kind that gets etched into ones memory.

We called my doctor who said, to relax and that he will see me later. Later kept coming and so did the contractions, every 10 minutes. They weren't getting any stronger just longer. The doctor had asked us to come back closer to home at this time, feeling that the contractions were going to kick in soon and that I may not make it back.

We left the kids with the family and proceeded home. By the time my brother in law brought the kids back we were still home and going nowhere. I called the doctor around 9 pm and said that I was hungry, what could I eat. I missed the bar-b-que and needed something to give me a little strength. He told me what I was allowed to have and that was the last time I spoke to him that night.

I ate and then went to sleep. I did not wake until morning. Somehow I was able to sleep through all the contractions. When I called the doctor, he asked where I was, so I told him in bed. It had already been over twelve hours and he needed to see me immediately.

So, in the not thinking manner which is common to people in labor, I drove myself to the doctor while my husband stayed home and waited for his parents who had expected us to call all night long. When I arrived at the doctor's office, I went to the desk and signed in.

"What are you doing, get in here, you're in labor." I looked up, it was the doctor.

It was time for my first ultrasound. They needed to see just what was going on. Sure enough my little one had completely turned around. They did not want to try and turn the baby because all of the umbilical cord was around the head of the baby and it was possible for the baby to turn into the umbilical cord, which would turn into a true emergency.

The doctor turned to me and said that they needed to do a cesarean section to get the baby out safely. I was horrified. I sat there and cried. My rational mind said, it was for the best and that I completely trusted the doctor. However, rational minds and labor don't always go hand and hand. The emotional part took over and said how after having a nine pound baby the natural way do I need a c-section?

My doctor was completely understanding, he waited there with me until he felt I was able to drive myself back home. He then had a nurse walk me out to the car. Still with some apprehension and nervousness I drove myself home to pick up my husband so we could go to the hospital. The drive home usually takes only 10 minutes, somehow at this moment it seemed to take an hour. The cars were whizzing by me and many thoughts were racing through my mind. Like, what the heck am I doing in this car right now. Is the baby ok? Did I do something wrong by falling asleep? How could I not tell that the baby turned? What was my husband going to think? Finally I pulled into the driveway.

When I walked into the front door my mother-in-law was coming in the side door. She gave me a really big smile of assurance, and a hug to match. My daughter stood there and then started to cry, "why is mommy crying? Is she ok?" It was at this point that I needed to keep my composure, if not for me at least for her. My mother-in-law was great, she scooped her up and off they went into the kitchen for a "special breakfast" as she told her.

My husband gathered my stuff and took this opportunity to leave without saying goodbye. He was more concerned that the baby was ok to even stop to think that I did anything wrong. I told him how I was feeling and he thought I was crazy.

I suppose that was exactly what I needed to hear, for it was then that I started concentrating on getting this baby out and not on myself. We walked into the hospital to see that everyone was ready for us. It is probably like this for those people who schedule their c-sections. Things were running like a well-oiled machine. We went from one place to another with precision timing. The nurses prepped me for surgery, with my intravenous fluids, my sedative and the anesthesiologist came to give me my epidural. Only this time the medicine was given not just to take the edge off my back but to put my entire lower half of my body asleep so that I could be awake for the procedure, yet feel nothing.

When my doctor came in to check me he asked why I had not felt any sudden or strong movement. I then reminded him, of which person he was dealing with. His response was, "oh, yeah the dancer." Referring to my baby.

As I lay on the table I hear a familiar voice, it was our pediatrician. It was their standard practice to come to the hospital for their patients in such an emergency. Of course, being the lunatic that I am, the first thought that went through my head was that now the doctor's office was backed up and it was my fault. I realized that I should have been happy to see him, although as I said before, the rational mind was not at work here.

During the entire procedure the doctor made sure he informed me of every step. When they opened me up he let us know that the baby was in no danger and that there apparently was plenty of room in there for the baby to have turned safely, we finally could exhale. Not a harrowing ordeal, however it did test ones endurance. Upon pulling the baby out the doctor told me not to worry about the epidural affecting the baby's alertness – this one was still dancing.

The dancer was here at last, all 8 pounds 14 ½ ounces of her.

The nurses waited until most of the epidural wore off before bringing me to my room. It was then that I was finally able to see this beauty. After a c-section you're in the hospital a little longer so my husband took this opportunity to bring the other ones up to see me. We had a happy 2 day old birthday party together. It was great, and a start of a whole new tradition. Dinner in the hospital with mommy and new baby.

Even at their tender ages of 2 and 3, they were so filled with unconditional love for this new addition in their lives. The true emotions that were felt when they were able to hold "their baby" was amazing. Their eyes lit up and their smiles were tremendous. My son had only one question, "do we get to take her home?"

Chapter 4

Happy New Year to us, we're going to have a baby. With the confirmation from the doctor, a new chapter in our lives has now begun. You may think it's just more of the same, however, my children seem to thrive on coming up with new things. New ways to make me feel, new places to bang against. But this time, no new doctor. The practice I was with last time proved to be remarkable in so many ways. I was lucky to find a group where I liked all the doctors that were a part of it.

So far we didn't find it too difficult to adjust to being outnumbered by our children, at least with this one we would both be carrying two at a time. These two will be 24 months apart, the good part about that is I was not going to have to purchase a double stroller. The first two walked quite well, and for long distances when necessary. The present baby will be 2 and most likely only need an umbrella stroller at that point. Knowing my kids, they will probably want to walk the baby themselves.

Although I had never used an ultrasound during pregnancy before, this one was going to be a little different because of the last one being a cesarean section. Plus, being that all of the other children were on the large side, the doctors wanted to monitor everything more closely so that the scar tissue wouldn't be disturbed. They were hoping for a smaller baby.

With the first ultrasound, the doctor noted that everything was moving in the right direction. The first 3 months flew by without any problems. There was very little nausea, and I can say with a smile that there were no growing pains either, if you know what I mean.

With each pregnancy I was very fortunate to be able to lose all my weight by the time the baby was 6 months old. Starting back at my original weight made a great difference to me psychologically. Knowing I was going to be gaining again. I did notice one thing though, that with each pregnancy I started showing physical signs of being pregnant earlier.

The hardest part of going through this particular pregnancy was that the doctors' wanted me to take the glucose test more than once. It's a test that is used to determine if you have gestational diabetes. It sounds like a serious condition, and can be if not detected or treated. Maybe my doctor was being a little over cautious but a little over is better than not enough.

My biggest problem with the test wasn't the test itself but that I found that no matter what the flavor was, the liquid they ask you to drink is horrid. It could be because I hate sweet things, I also don't care for seltzer and this liquid is pretty much a combination of those two tastes. At least to me. Then they go and flavor it orange, which would just put me over the edge—I personally despise orange soda.

The other hard thing was going through the whole summer getting larger and larger. It's hard to stay cool when you are pregnant regardless of the time of year, so you can understand that the prospect of going through another summer pregnant didn't rank high on the thrills meter.

Besides there is only so much you can take off when you are hot.

I had to keep drinking for fear of dehydrating. Why was I so afraid? Well for one thing I was so darn sweaty from the heat. Not that you can dehydrate from sweat but from someone who doesn't sweat much at all – it was a change I wasn't ready for. So I basically spent the last trimester of the pregnancy either drinking, going to the bathroom or doing the laundry (because you know I had to change cloths a lot too). Let's not forget the four hundred showers I felt that I was taking too. My skin was not very appreciative.

So I tried to use lotion, only to find that the smell of it made me sick. The last trimester didn't seem like a great time to start throwing up. So I let the skin go without too much adverse affects.

Remember me saying that each child brought something new? Well, this baby was having a field day with banging around. It wasn't kicking or rolling or anything like that, it truly was banging. First, there was a soft movement, then

49

BANG! Right in my ribs. If I didn't know better I would think that the baby was picking up a hand or foot and banging me with full force. So much so that by the end of my eighth month my ribs were tender to touch.

This is a real problem when you have other children who still want mommy to pick the up and who still love to jump on top of me for a hug. The doctor said the baby probably bruised a rib. When I asked what I could do about it, he smiled and said, "Give birth." It really made life hard knowing that to hug my other children would set my eyes rolling and sometimes a tear or two flowing. I just kept telling myself this too shall pass.

Soon after my 9th month began, I was visited by frequent false labors. A false labor can feel like the real thing, only it stops after an hour or so. At this time the false labors would come about two or three a week and were lasting in upwards of 3 hours. I was told by a couple of people to try and drink a small glass of wine to "test" if it was real or false, if it stopped it was false, if not call the doctor. This thought did not appeal to me too much so I never bothered asking the doctor what he thought.

Trying to sleep through this wasn't easy. I knew all these false labors would pay off eventually, I just didn't know that it would last until a week *after* my due date. Funny how I always thought that each child was supposed to get earlier and/or faster. There's another myth that was proven wrong by my kids.

In fact, we had company one week and I kept running into them in the middle of the night—racing each other for the bathroom. Each time they would say—"Now?" and I would just laugh and say—no, baby is just bouncing on the bladder.

My due date was around the same time as the last child. This made me crazy, I really didn't' want the children to have the same birthday. After all, they weren't twins. The down side was that I was not sure that I was going to have much of a choice in the matter. As the date came closer my anxiety grew. Rationally speaking it was kind of selfish of me, who was I to say when each child was to be born? Many people have the same birthday as younger siblings. Most people handle it with great maturity, I guess I wasn't one of them. Something about it just bothered me.

The night before my soon-to-be 2 year old's birthday I sat down. I did nothing all evening except keep my legs up and relax. I purposely did a lot of nothing the next day as well. After dinner I decided that by the time this next child would be born it would be the next day so I got up and took care of everything that needed to be done. Little did I know that it would be another 3 days before I went into labor. Do you think resting helped? I'm not sure one hundred percent but at the very least it made me feel better. Sometimes that's the most important part. Don't ever forget to take care of your own needs too while you're running and doing everything for everyone else.

The labor with this one was rather simple. Around mid-day I began having some contractions but they seemed sporadic, I first realized this one was not false by the intensity of it and by the fact that the baby must have dropped some because that rib was no longer being hit. I finally went to the hospital around 5 or 6 in the evening.

The doctor's were still concerned about the scar from the cesarean section I just had and how it would weather another birth. This little one had other plans though, just because it looked as if I was moving along at a relatively quick pace doesn't mean the baby wanted to come out. It looked like it was going to be another long one. So my husband pulled up a chair and sat down.

When you are in labor your legs are up in stirrups, your body on an incline so that your belly seems to be right between your thighs. It was night time so the window in the room was dark. Here I was feeling my belly being contracted my head seemed to be pounding and for some odd reason I just wanted some good old fashion comfort. There was this overwhelming desire to be held myself, the kind of feeling you get as a child when you don't know why but you just need someone to hold you. That in mind it was time to push the baby out. I remember looking all over the room for that source of comfort. I then looked longingly out the darken window. There it was, as plain as the nose on my face, an image of my grandmother whispering to me that everything was going to be alright.

By now you probably think I am a total lunatic, however, when I spoke to a friend of mine, who works in the psychiatric field, afterwards they told me they felt there was nothing wrong with me. Just as people say that they saw their whole life flash before them in times of great danger, my subconscious flashed a vote of confidence to me.

We all search for that certain something that will calm us down in times of anxiety. There are people who put "good luck" things in their pockets when going on an interview. People who are in the hospital long term who like to surround themselves with pieces of home or fond memories. No, I wasn't crazy, I probably did see just what I wanted and/or needed to.

This baby was bent on hanging around up there and decided that a few extra pushes were necessary. It wasn't until 11:00 that night that the head finally showed itself. What a big head it was indeed. The doctor was so impressed that I did not tear getting this baby's head out. I needed only two small stitches but that was all. Having the head out was the hard part with this baby.

One more push and the rest of the baby came flying out. Big head yet a long and skinny body.

Weighing in at 8lb 8oz she was a beauty.

The doctor mentioned to me that during the time of banging it was probably when the baby was trying to turn it's head down. Considering the size of her head he's not surprised that I was bruised, nor was he surprised that it took a long time for her to get in position.

That said, and baby checked, the doctor smiled and left us to enjoy our newest bundle of joy.

Chapter 5

Believe it or not we were just as excited to find out we were expecting our fifth child as when we found out we were expecting our first. To realize the multitude of things that can go awry during pregnancy, makes each one all that much more special. Each time we were able to conceive also reminds of how lucky we are, when there are so many in this world who either can not, or can't without a lot of medicinal help. We know in our hearts that we truly have been blessed.

At the point of the pregnancy that we were telling people I received a lot of uncalled for comments. "Still trying for another boy, huh?" that was the most annoying. "Don't you have enough" was a good one. But the one that was the best actually came from my own grandmother, "Well, honey, I can't exactly stand over your bed to tell you to stop." At least her comment was followed by a "take could care of yourself".

My true friends were happy for us. The ones who were not, well, I don't know if there is an explanation for it. Some people acted as if it meant a harder burden on them. When I was seen at the mall or park with all my kids, total strangers would feel compelled to comment. As if it was there business to do so. After awhile I just learned to let people talk and then politely walk away.

There was obviously a lot more going on in my life during this pregnancy. We had carpool, bus stops, and homework, plus all the other things that needed to get done on a daily basis. Being busy never bothered me.

During the beginning of this pregnancy, when I was around 10 weeks pregnant, I was sitting down playing with my older kids when, boom, this flush of warm liquid came out of me. I ran directly to the bathroom not knowing what I was about to see—as it turned out all I saw was blood – everywhere. Needless to say, I freaked out. The first call was to my husband because it would take him the longest to get home from where he worked. The second was to the doctor.

It was with a reassuring voice that I was told, chances were good things were going to work out, but just the same I needed to get to the doctor's office as soon as I could. I had to wait for carpool to come home first. I gathered up the kids and off we went. Due to all my confusion I neglected to find a place to bring them. When I walked in with everyone, the nurses couldn't get over it. They never saw them all together and were just loving all the wonderful shades of blonde on top of their heads.

The kids thought it was funny to hide behind the curtain in the examination room. You know the curtain, the one which you go behind to change before an exam. It was just big enough for them to hide in. I think all their giggling kept me calm. The doctor had to do a new type of ultrasound, this one was an internal one to see just what was going on more precisely.

After a thorough exam the doctor determined that things would be fine. His only instruction was to lay low for a couple of days and not to pick up anyone.

Easy for him to say, how was I to get everyone into the car? Say no more, they sent a nurse out to help me. Then he said, go home and sit down. That's it, I was not supposed to do anything else for 2 days. Thankfully this was a Friday, so my husband was going to be home for these two days of me doing absolutely nothing. Hard to do as a mother of 4.

The kids took this opportunity to snuggle with mom. One of them was always by my side the entire weekend. They thought they were helping me. It was good for me that the doctor said only 2 days, because that amount of close love can make a person seriously claustrophobic.

My friends and neighbors were great too. They brought meals over before Friday night was even over. Having a strong support circle is what helped me get this far in the first place. We are always there for each other no matter how little or how big.

With the events of the trauma over, the next few months went quickly and uneventfully by. The greatest activity of my children's evening was, to see how many things the baby will kick off mommy's stomach. It wasn't so bad when only one person was putting things there, but can you imagine what it looked like when all 4 were putting things on me? It became a race to see whose toy would last the longest. They were really happy to 'play" with the baby. So I had to muster up the patience to let them do it, I didn't want them to feel I was pushing them away because of the new baby.

As you can imagine, there were many things going on in the house besides the pregnancy. We were re-doing a couple of the kids bedrooms. The color of the room could not be determined until the baby was born. If it was a boy then my son would get the larger room and share with the baby, if it was a girl than the last girl born would be sharing with the baby. The anticipation caused a little friction now and then, but we mulled through it.

Sometimes my son would get very angry at me saying I didn't want him to have a brother. This was hard to deal with at times. One time I even mentioned it to the pediatrician and had him talk to my son on one of his visits. It was obvious that he was trying to say it wasn't up to mommy to decide, however, in the eyes of a six year old, and I quote, "if it's in mommy than it's her fault." Neither the doctor nor myself could counter act that child's logic. For him it made perfect sense, it's her body therefore – it's her fault. There was only so much information that we wanted to give a six-year old. For good or bad, that is what when we decided to stop.

We were finally able to get him to understand that boy or girl he was loved in his own right and it wouldn't matter what the baby was. We explained to him that this baby was going to add lots of love and fun to the whole family. He seemed to understand it, although I can't say that he accepted it.

In any event, the pregnancy was going well. Having been in my last trimester in the warmer weather for the rest of the kids left me with little to wear in January and February for this one. I was due in March.

Knowing how large our family was already, I really did not want to be buying too much at this point. So I found a few things and just layered them when it was cold. It didn't look so great but at least it was something. I actually bought some large shirts in the men's department. Believe it or not the shirts were cut to be big in all the places I needed it to be.

My life was so busy by the time I was pregnant this time that I feel a lot of those minor discomforts and other physical problems I had in the past either didn't bother me enough to notice or didn't happen. This pregnancy like the last one, went by with relative ease. I for one was extremely thankful.

Then that fateful Friday came, the usual morning routine, lunches, breakfast, getting everyone ready for work and school. I didn't feel right but I knew I had an appointment at 10 in the morning so I didn't feel compelled to call the doctor right away. My husband told me he was going to be in a meeting at that time, so if I was in labor to call him at the meeting.

Don't misunderstand me, we don't approach having a baby as routine, it's just that I didn't need him at that moment and I had an appointment in a couple of hours anyway. No point in making an emergency out of something that was not one.

By the time I saw the doctor I was definitely in labor. He told me to go home and get myself ready. So, I went home, finished cooking dinner, did some laundry, and oh yeah, called my husband and told him to come home around 3 pm. I figured I was playing the odds that this one wasn't going to move too fast either. Then I called my mother-in-law who worked only 10 minutes away to have her come around 3 as well.

My own brother called in the meantime and I told him everyone was coming home around 3 and I'll probably go then. Three o'clock came and so did my husband, his mother and my brother all within 5 minutes of each other. My husband busied himself with bathing the kids and finishing up dinner. I had to remind him that that is why his mother was here, and that it was time to go.

Oops! Forgot why he was home. Once he was refocused, we were on our way to the hospital the nurse recognized us from one of the previous births. What I found even more impressive was that she remembered that my kids don't drop during pregnancy and that I usually needed additional help from the drug patosin.

By this time the maternity ward had changed so much I didn't even recognize the place. They now had LDRP rooms (labor, delivery, recovery and postpartum all in one room). The rooms you gave birth in were also the rooms you recovered in and stayed in until you went home. They looked like a hotel room. You had your own bathroom, the mother-to-be's bed which changed from a regular looking bed to a birthing bed, a couch-like chair for your coach and the baby's bassinet was fixed on top of a set of drawers. The drawers had all the essentials you would need for your baby; diapers, cleaning cloths, a change of clothes, a supply of 4oz bottles of formula and an extra receiving blanket to swaddle the baby in.

The décor was done in soothing light wood tones with a floral border around the top of the room. There was a television hooked up high so that while you were lying down you didn't have to do much to see it. Some hotels don't even give you so much space.

You had another choice too, either keep the baby in your room or send the baby back to the nursery if you wanted some sleep. Not feeling like you are in a sterile hospital room made the whole experience much nicer. The truth is there are very few times other than giving birth that a person actually wants to be in the hospital.

Now that I was set up in this "hotel" maybe an hour had passed. We were both assuming that this baby was going to take awhile as did the others. It was nice to be proved wrong for once. With only a very little epidural, before I knew it, it was time to push. Three pushes later and only 2 hours after we had arrived, the baby was born.

Pushing this one out was not so hard at all. The head was completely bald and as round as a cue ball. Only this cue ball was smiling back at you.

Weighing in at 8lb 8oz and, thankfully, the picture of health.

When I came home from the hospital I had a rash all over my face, it looked as if I was sunburned. Turns out I had "fifth disease".

Thankfully, the baby did not get it—only my oldest daughter did. Funny, you went into the hospital "healthy" and come home with more than just a baby.

It is really just a virus, but it did put a little strain on everyone who wanted to come close to mommy. They hadn't seen me for a while and didn't understand why they could not be all over me as they had done before.

As I mentioned before, my son was having some amount of difficulty with this pregnancy. However, when you have a 6 year old boy who sees he already has 3 other sisters, having another one became a real problem in the family. It is not easy for a child to understand why he is the only one who has a room all to himself and everyone else gets to share a room with someone. As opposed to looking at it that he doesn't have to share, his perception was that he was being pushed aside.

This became a source of tremendous anxiety for him. It also was the cause of many fights between him and I. Questions like, "Why don't you want to give me a brother?" came up quite often. Comments such as, "I promise I will be good to him, I'll teach him how to play ball and share my toys" were also part of frequent conversations.

It was at this point that we had to look for some outside help. I contacted the pediatrician once again who took the time out to speak to my son in an informal setting. He also gave me a name of a social worker who might be able to teach me ways to communicate better so that he will understand that it was ok to be angry. This person was very helpful. But the best help came from the baby herself.

She endeared herself to him all the way from his head down to his toes. It was my son who could calm her down just by picking her up. It was he who could always get her to laugh, and to top things off it was his name that she learned how to pronounce first – right after daddy of course. She gave him the total unconditional love that he needed. Many times she would fall asleep on him while he sat on the couch and he wouldn't even get up so as not to disturb her.

In the end things turned out well, I don't know if it would for everyone but we are thankful that it did for us.

Chapter 6

My husband and I have been very blessed with the ability to have children with only the equipment that God has provided. My pregnancies went the gamut from basic complaints to more serious ones. As it turned out all of my deliveries were as different as my children's personalities. The one in which I would like to draw your attention to the most, however, is the last one.

The majority of the world thinks that women carry babies and deliver them as a matter of course. After all it's been going on for centuries now. One thing that still remains a mystery to some people is how women used to die during childbirth. There are a multitude of people who assume it was the doctors fault, and still others feel it was somehow something the woman did herself. On the contrary, often times things happen that are a total surprise to all parties concerned.

This pregnancy was different in countless ways from the beginning. Although we never had much trouble conceiving, this time we did. It took us quite a long time in comparison to the others. In fact we were already getting worried. I know it may seem silly because we already had a large family, but things are all relative. Going from having trouble conceiving you expect the next time to be the same. However, going from conceiving with ease to having almost a full year of trying seemed like cause for concern. At least this is one thing you don't mind working hard at to achieve.

It has been my experience, of either my own pregnancies or that of my friends, that morning sickness usually lasts no longer than the first trimester. With this child it completely took me over. I was sick morning, noon, or night with these incredible almost flu-like feeling for almost a complete 5 months.

Many of my favorite foods became unappetizing to me as well. As the weeks went by my body was feeling more and more sluggish. The doctor kept on saying it was because I was taking care of so many more people now. I am sure that was a strong factor in the situation, however, it was a different sort of tired, one I never had experienced with the others. There even were times when I needed to rest before midday. The need was so strong it would overtake me until I would actually sit and/or lay down for half an hour or so.

I went in for my check-up at around 39 weeks to have a discussion about my condition, both physical and emotional. Together my doctor and I came to the conclusion to go ahead and set a date to induce me.

On the morning we went to the hospital everything was to be going according to schedule. Once again, I was set up in and LDRP room. Did I mention that you get your own bathroom? I don't even have one of those at home. It's a great atmosphere. The hospital staff enjoys it as well, the whole feel of the place puts you in a different frame of mind then that of a hospital.

But I digress once again. As my labor progressed things continued to have the appearance of a normal delivery. My water broke, the contractions came at a steady pace, everything seemed to be progressing quite normally. Before we knew it, the morning had passed and the time came to push the baby out.

First push came without too much difficulty on my part. The second one, on the other hand, seemed to wipe me out completely. Me head felt light and my arms felt weak, nothing about me felt as it should at that moment. I made an announcement to the doctor that I could not go on. I felt faint. Within 10 seconds a whole team came rushing in, they had lost the baby's heartbeat on the monitor, a second nurse was putting another IV in my other arm.

Just as I was about to pass out I got a glance of my husband's face. His hand was over his mouth and his eyes said, "Oh my God what's going on" I had never seen him so scared. He looked so completely terrified.

The next thing I knew I was being flipped upside down. They had me strapped into the bed and my feet were in the air, and my head was down. I do remember fearing I was going to fall out of the bed onto my head. My head heard words and commotion but my eyes were not open, I could not see who was doing what. No matter how hard I tried to open my eyes during all this, they just wouldn't.

I have to admit that during all this time I completely forgot that I was trying to have a baby and was just trying to wake up. Hearing people call you and hearing the bells and whistles of a hospital room, yet not seeing them was beginning to scare me in a way I had never known before. I was in a darkness yet I felt part of me was aware of my surroundings only I wasn't sure exactly where my surroundings were.

As I came to they lifted me slowly back into an upright position. The baby's heart rate was found and it was still my turn to push. The doctor looked a little worried and asked if I thought I could push anymore. They were prepared to do another c-section if I was unable to handle a natural birth.

I remember saying yes, although I wasn't sure how. My arms felt like wet noodles, my head was still in a daze, and I didn't even feel the baby anymore – only an incredible pain across my chest area, right under my ribs. I truly feel that my strength at that time came straight from an angle because there was nothing left in me. Then, with only one or two more pushes this beautiful gift from God appeared – unharmed.

Unfortunately, I was so physically wiped out that I could not even lift my head to see her, they had to prop me up. My husband was so elated he didn't know who to kiss first. The entire room was filled with genuine emotions and a lot of them.

It was then that this feeling of severe pressure near my lower ribs became more intense. Everyone seemed to feel that it was from the trauma of being flipped, and that maybe the baby hit me in the process. The doctor said I was probably going to need more rest than usual to recover from this delivery, and that they would keep a close eye on me.

When things calmed down a bit my husband and I finally were able to look at the time. Why was this important? Well, we actually had an appointment with someone that afternoon that could not be rearranged. The doctor assured him that I really just needed a little rest. It was normal, people can pass out during the pushing process. We made a group decision that it was ok for him to go to the meeting, then go home and bring the others up to see their new sister.

Once he left the doctor checked me over once again, the baby was being checked by the pediatrician and the nurse was sitting down to do some of the post pardom paperwork. Some part of me made me ask the nurse to stay awhile because I wasn't feeling right. There was something about my body as a whole that just wasn't jiving with me. She was more than happy to stay.

The pains and intense pressure I felt in my chest never subsided, so along with the discomforts of giving birth I had this to contend with. I could not get comfortable at all. Just as things were at a calm, I called over to the nurse to say, I was not well, before I knew it I had passed out again. This time, however, I heard nothing. I was down for the count.

When I opened my eyes there seemed to be a dozen people in my room again. Maybe I was seeing double, who knows, but there was a multitude of people in there. The doctor checked my chest area again and this time called for an ultrasound to be brought up.

One thing the doctor had mentioned to me before the baby was born was that as you have more children, you stand a greater risk of bleeding too much after birth. This was not the case, in fact at this point the doctor restated that she did not remember seeing much blood at all.

For those of you who have ever had an ultrasound, you know that the technician doesn't put much pressure on you at all. Under these circumstances I had so much discomfort from the pressure and pain that I felt as if a hot brick was being pushed around on me by a 500 pound hand. The technician kept apologizing even though we both knew he was being as gentle as possible.

As I looked around the room, everybody had the same look on their face – that of concern and worry. Not what you want to see in a room full of doctors and nurses. The doctor told me they saw internal bleeding and that I had lost a lot of blood already, which is why I had passed out, again.

Surgery was a must. There were two distinct possibilities, one was that my previous cesarean scar opened – in which case they would try to repair it, or that my uterus burst in which case it would have to come out. Either way at that moment I was not in a position to bargain.

My husband had not gotten back yet, so believe it or not they had me sign the release papers. I wonder what that signature looks like? I always joke around now thinking if it could really be legible or even legal?

They immediately laid me down and rushed me down the corridor to the operating room. A friend of mine had come up to see me and the baby, she was the first to witness what was going on. I am not sure the doctor had even been in touch with my husband yet.

I remember going down the corridor, into the elevator and feeling absolutely every small bump there was to feel. My insides were so sensitive that even the floor seams felt as if they were the size of speed bumps. Upon seeing the operating room, the doctor introduced herself to me as if I really didn't know who she was, maybe I didn't. There was a second doctor that was there as an assistant. I also remember the anesthesiologist speaking to me in a calm voice yet, for some reason, I found myself fighting with the her. She said to me in a very soothing way that she was putting an oxygen mask over me, and yet in my wearied state I still tried fighting. I never asked why, I am sure there is some rational reason for it. Or not.

Picture yourself in my husband's shoes, how he must have felt to get this phone call, "Excuse me sir this is the hospital calling, your wife who just had a baby is being rushed into emergency surgery."

I was always told that a person's hemoglobin is supposed to be around 12-14, mine was down to 4. I needed 4 units of blood. My uterus had burst after all, one of the doctors told my friend that it looked like a blown out tire, and that she was happy that the baby did not try to get out through that hole, it was that big.

In recovery my husband came in and I just kept apologizing. Obviously there was nothing to apologize for, I just didn't know what else to say.

In the ICU they had brought me the baby and let me try to nurse her. With both arms being nice and bruised up from all the IV's and with my present state of "strength" this was next to an impossible task. The pain was too much and I had to stop. Being postpartum is one thing, but this was an intensity I never knew a person could feel. They wheeled the baby back up to the nursery. Rationally, I knew it was the right thing to do, emotionally I was torn apart.

I was in ICU for almost 48 hours. The baby was born Friday around mid afternoon, and I was in surgery by 5 pm. I was not able to get back to my LDRP room until Sunday morning.

The people transferring me from ICU back upstairs were not very helpful, in getting me from one bed to another. They had expected me to do it on my own. Imagine that. I could barely lift my arms to give myself a piece of ice and they wanted me to lift my entire body up and over onto another bed. Stars weren't the only thing I was seeing at that time.

The LDRP rooms have a bed that the bottom half detaches when the stirrups need to come out. Because of the surgery my doctor ordered a whole bed for me. This time the nurses made sure to help me. They were shocked to hear of my first experience, and assured me that the people moving me the first time probably didn't know what had happened. In fact one of the nurses went to investigate, I never found out the results of that but I guess it didn't really matter much.

My husband brought the kids by, as was our usual tradition in the hospital, only this time I could not see them. Or should I say, I didn't want them to see me. I still had the two IV's in and other things. Besides I was ashen in color. Not a pretty picture for young kids. It was very hard to send them away but I knew I had to. My husband wanted them to spend time with the baby though, so they took the baby in a nearby, unused room to say hi to her. I do remember hearing them giggle and sing happy birthday to her.

Sunday night came and the nurse was trying to get me to eat so that I would be able to take oral medication and not in the IV. I barely was able to eat one quarter of the roll. It took all my strength to eat anything at all. The bread felt as hard as a leather to chew. When my friend took over in trying to feed me, the nurse left. Shortly after, my friend left too. The effort of chewing was too much for me.

Almost 48 hours after giving birth I had only seen the baby a few minutes. I called to the nurse's station to have her brought back to me. I was feeling conscious enough to have her in my room. As the nurse brought her in she began to wake. We tried nursing one more time. Although it was quite painful to hold her, I just really needed to. The nurse stayed with me to help because I was not in any condition to get up to change her. She put her back on me but I could bear no more pressure on my belly so she put her back to sleep. We both decided it would be best for the baby to stay in the nursery one more night.

Once again a decision was proven correct. Around 9pm I had to ring the nurse again. I was so nauseated I didn't know what to do with myself. They gave me some water to sip and something to calm it down. It did not. To most people I know throwing up actually makes them feel better. Me, it terrifies. Unbeknownst to me, my worst nightmare was about to come true. I felt as if there was a volcano churning inside me.

When the next shift of nurses made their rounds to introduce themselves they said their name and asked how I felt. Normal so far. Only my response came by way of the most horrific projectile vomiting I'd every known. My stitches were being pulled on so hard I was afraid my whole stomach was going to open up. When it all subsided I found myself once again in a room full of people. Nurses cleaning me up, janitors cleaning off floors, other nurses changing my bedding (with me still in the bed) and finally the doctor to make sure the stitches did not open in any way, and to make sure there were no other issues.

Already feeling as if a semi truck had been pulled out of me in two directions simultaneously. Having absolutely no physical strength left I had only my spiritual strength to keep me afloat. With all that was going on, this was not what I would call a normal delivery.

The night was very long considering I slept all of 10 minutes. When morning actually did come, so did whatever was left inside of me. I felt as if I was beginning to be a real pest to the nurses but what else could I do – so I buzzed them again. They came in right away, along with the doctor who sent me right away for an X-ray to make sure everything was intact. Things were as they should, the decision was to put me on a liquid diet for at least 24-36 hours.

When Tuesday morning came I was finally able to hold the baby and nurse her without my IV's in. I was also finally able to eat real food. Even hospital food can taste good after not eating anything at all for 4 days.

The next day and a half was spent getting my physical strength back and improving my hemoglobin.

I was discharged on Thursday. Spending 6 days in a hospital for childbirth, when most of the time you are lucky if your insurance pays for 48 hours. The discharging doctor was very specific in his instructions. We discussed that I had better abide by these conditions or my 4-month recovery will take close to a year.

This kind of time frame was bizarre to me. I have always bounced back within days of having a baby – now he says months? It was at this time that my doctor also had some assurances for me. These events had nothing to do with having a large family, it had nothing to do with being induced, it simply had to do with how this particular pregnancy was handled by my body.

To think that as little as 20 years ago I may not have made it home with my baby. She would have gone home only with her father. I am thankful for the technological advances the medical world has done.

Getting pregnant, pregnancy, and especially childbirth are not things that should be taken lightly. Writing this is not meant to make anyone afraid of childbirth, it is written to make you aware that even with all the technological advances we do have today to save your life, it doesn't prevent the doctors from having to use them. The difference is, now we can have many, many more happier endings.

Chapter 7
What do I do now?

Before I let you go, I just wanted to talk about a few more things. Naming a child, for instance, can be easy for some and yet it can bring complete turmoil to others.

It is our family's tradition to name a child after someone who has died. Many people feel it is an honor to have someone named after them within the first year of them being gone.

That was the case with our first child. Unfortunately for my husband his grandmother had died shortly after we were married. As far as we were concerned the girl's name was automatically going to be hers. My family on the other hand had a different opinion. They felt that the bride's side of the family got the first name.

My statement to them was that I am no longer a bride, I am a mother-to-be. Their rebuttal? If it's a boy, it had better be named from their family. Meanwhile, my husband and I were just wishing for a healthy child, boy or girl made no difference to us.

The second child again was a source of argument. While my son was still in the hospital, we did not know when he was coming home, and my parents called to talk about the name they wanted.

It was then that we decided that whatever we will be naming our children will be up to us. We will not reveal what names we are thinking of because the aggravation that comes with it, wasn't worth it.

Not all families will have this problem. In the event that you do, try to keep your composure, it is not worth losing family ties over. One must always remember that you are not arguing over a what, but over a person, it's not the christening of a boat.

Now you are a mother

Some of my most frequently asked question is, "how do you do it?"

Even a mother of one knows that many things change about your life when you have a baby. Especially if you are nursing, you are on someone else's time schedule.

You not only are responsible for feeding this person but you are responsible for everything that person needs – along with your own schedule.

A decision my husband and I made together was that we didn't want to run our lives based on the baby's schedule. We wanted to make sure that the baby's schedule fit into ours. The baby can sleep wherever we would need to be, and feeding would be just as easy wherever we were.

Especially while I was nursing exclusively – there was nothing to bring. With the increased availability of bottled water and powdered formula – a baby's bottle can be made fresh anywhere you go. There are even insulated bottle holders so that you can keep your water pre-warmed.

Learning how to prioritize has helped me immensely. Whether to run to the phone or pick up the mess the baby just spilled, whether to run to get the oven buzzer or finish changing the baby's diaper. Your day becomes filled with these types of "problems".

Remember one quick thing, the phone can wait. With the availability of caller-identification on most phones now, it is easy to call back the person who just called, or let the answering machine pick up, most things can wait the two minutes it takes to get yourself better situated to talk on the phone.

If the baby is safe in his/her crib or playpen, go ahead take the food out of the oven, answer the door.

Those two extra minutes of crying won't hurt the baby, especially if they can see you from where they are.

One other thing I found very helpful was that I took my kids with me all the time. It didn't bother me to shop with them or run errands with them. I tried very hard not to be tied down to their schedule but to make them part of my schedule. Let me rephrase that, I tried very hard to make the children a part of my life — not the other way around.

It is my opinion that by doing so they learned how to behave in a public. They learned how to stay near me and when it was time to go further. Helping mommy became fun for them. To this day they don't feel that running errands is a heavy chore.

Organization is the tool I have used. It is the best thing you can have on your side. It's also the only thing you have full control over.

Having someone who works with you is good too, whether that someone is your husband or just a support group of friends either way will help you. Don't think you have to go this alone, you didn't get here alone.

Making time for yourself will help give you that recoup time that so many new mothers need. Sometimes, instead of running around and trying to get things done while the baby is sleeping, sit down and have a tall drink with a good book.

Then when the baby wakes up you are ready to be with him/her again. You're no longer totally stressed.

Remembering mommy is the hardest thing to do, but the most vital. After the cord is cut you are no longer "tied to the baby". You are allowed to be yourself.

Stop, look at your day and figure out how best to accommodate both you and the baby. If getting a sitter or going with a friend is what will help, than do so. Don't let guilt get in your way of rational thinking. Don't get me wrong, there will be times when your day is totally dedicated to the baby. The hard part is not to let it overwhelm you in the process. Sometimes it's helpful to think of what you will accomplish in the whole week, this way by the end of the week if your whole list is crossed off you know you did well. If one day or a couple half days were completely tied up with the baby you know that you still have tomorrow to get something done.

Not everything can be pushed off to the next day, so thinking hard and trying to prioritize each day before you start is a good goal to have.

You'll be a good mother, you will love the baby with more emotion you knew you had in you, and you will figure it out. Trusting your instincts, having self-confidence, and believing in what you are doing is right for your situation and your baby will help you get through the rough times.

Yes, there will be rough times. During those times where you feel you just want to scream and/or pull your hair out. Do it! Grab a nearby pillow and scream into it. Get the negative energy out, then go look at the baby whose eyes sparkle like dew on the top of a blade of grass, inhale...exhale...and pick the baby up. Once you are calm on the inside, you will see that the baby will respond more positively.

I found that the more agitated I was the crankier the babies were. They somehow can sense your nervousness. Actually, there were times when I would purposely nurse the baby through these times. It forced me to sit down and relax and it usually helped the baby as well. Other times, I would sit down with whomever was in the house and watch a video tape or play a game. Taking the time out of my reality and putting myself into theirs would get my mind off whatever it was that was bothering me. Sure I eventually had to get up and be an adult, but I was able to do it better when my inner energy level was in check.

Find what works for you—you will. If calling home is what works for you—then do that too. (sometimes anyway). My grandmothers were a tremendous source of good advice. Sure sometimes I felt it was outdated, but the basic principles are there. The biggest ingredient in their special potion? Unending love.

There is someone for everyone out there. As I said before, don't go it alone, you didn't get here that way don't expect to carry on that way.

Do I have any advice on bottle feeding?

Obviously going cold turkey from nursing was a bad idea, so when my son was born, we immediately tried a different method. The first bottle my son got was after he was a month old. My husband started giving him the night bottle before we put him down for the night. Our logic?

We didn't want the baby dependant on me to fall asleep. Formula, I'm told, is also heavier and can last longer, so why not do it at night? It gave me a break and it created a wonderful bond with my husband. We continued this method with the rest of the kids as well.

Once the babies were receiving a regular bottle, it wasn't as big of a deal to wean them off. The next bottle was determined by what was most convenient for my husband and also what would give the best relief for me. If you are a person who works out of the house your needs would vary greatly from a person working at home. The best thing to do is asses the needs of your household and wean accordingly. Many people I know saved one particular time for last because it was the time they enjoyed being with the baby the most. You may find you have a particular point of the day that works for you as well.

Once the baby is completely finished nursing you will still have a couple of days where your breasts may be tender, but it won't be too bad. I was always told to wear a tighter bra for those couple of days.

Burping?

Oh yeah. How do you get that baby to burp without coughing up the entire bottle they just drank? My first one was great, two little taps on the back and there came the gas. My son, of course, had to be difficult. My mother-in-law showed me how to move his legs around as if he was on a bicycle. Also, you can try gently pushing their knees to their chest, anything to move the gas bubble around. When you do hold the baby against you, remember the burping towel for your shoulder. You might want to make sure that the towel goes down a few inches in the back too. Babies are not neat when the burp something up.

Is it hard? No. I think I mentioned this before, and if I haven't I should have, the best advice I can give you about your baby is to learn who they are. What is good for one baby may not work on another, even if they are siblings.

Sleeping techniques, burping positions, feeding preferences, all seem like pretty routine things. However, if you don't know the baby in which you are dealing with and you are trying to do "what worked before" you may be surprised.

Babies are always changing, always growing, and hopefully always learning. The learning is not just for the babies. Just when you think you have the baby's schedule figured out, they go and change when and where they like to sleep. Don't panic, they will find a new routine, and this one may even be better than the first.

Babies in general

It will amaze and astound you just how dependant your little one is on you. You will take a step back and appreciate all that you are able to do when you see all that a baby has to learn. From holding its head up, or even holding onto your finger. When that first sounds of "baby talk" come out, and they way they have to learn how to use their tongue the right way.

All these subtle milestones, as well as the big ones like rolling over, crawling, holding a bottle by themselves, climbing a step and let's not forget the big one – walking, will bring you much joy and laughter and probably a few bumps and bruises too along the way. Don't worry, they will recover faster than you. It will be alright, you *can* do this.

Is parenting tough? Well, yes quite frankly it is. Would you have wanted to bring you up? You will learn as you go along, just like the rest of us have. You will continue to learn new things as each new stage of life comes up. There are no hard and fast rules for dealing with babies, children, adolescence or anything beyond that. Talk with people, get suggestions and then find what works in your particular situation. If you don't know who to call in a specific situation, try your pediatrician. They can be a wealth of information.

I hope I have shed some light on what you are about to get yourself into, or what you are in the midst of. If for any reason at any point of this book I insulted you or frightened you in any way than I sincerely apologize. That was not my intension.

I have heard from many people that a child will forget the pain they went through during teething, just as a woman forgets the pain she went through during childbirth. As I see my babies turn into teenagers I realized that the time has passed ever so quickly, yet in all honestly, my memories of the happy parts far outweigh those of the pain.

My hat is off to you, anyone who is expecting or trying, may your pregnancy come quickly, and your birthing experience be as calm as a gentle breeze. As all should go well so that you may be able to create your own glorious family memories. Be well.

Sincerely,

A mother of 6

About the Author

Teri Hirsch grew up in Missouri, at 21 she married and moved to New Jersey. She has always been in love with the power of the written word. Teri Hirsch speaks through her heart, which enables her to express her opinion of real life situations clearly and precisely. She speaks to you in a friendly tone from a person whose background is "been there, done that", not from a so-called "professional". Most importantly, her writing makes you feel that she is talking to you personally, as any good friend should.

www.ingramcontent.com/pod-product-compliance
Lightning Source LLC
Chambersburg PA
CBHW030344290526
45785CB00004B/1598